Whispers of Time

Whispers of Time

Understanding the End-of-Life Timeline

Peter M. Abraham, BSN, RN

Whispers of Time
Understanding the End-of-Life Timeline
Copyright © 2024 Peter M. Abraham, BSN, RN

Contact Info: author@2abraham.com

Second Edition: September 2024

DEDICATION

This book is dedicated to my wife Laura, who has stood by and with me from the time of our wedding, which occurred when I was still working in information technology through the ins and outs of nursing school, including all my tears from being out of school for over thirty years, and throughout all the ups and downs of my nursing career.

Table of Contents

Introduction

I still remember my Parkinson's patient using her rolling walker to come up to me with an appointment planner. She placed the planner before me and asked me to write down the date and time. I looked at her curiously and asked if she meant my next visit, explaining that I could give her the date, but the time might vary. She replied, "No, I want you to write down the date and time of my death." Despite my efforts to keep a composed expression, I'm sure I looked shocked. I responded, "Only God knows the exact date and time; all I can do is estimate." She promptly and politely replied, "Maybe I need a more experienced hospice nurse."

One of the shared experiences for everyone working in hospice, especially nurses, is being asked by patients, "When will I die?" or "How much longer do I have to live?" Family members often ask, "How long do they have to live?" and "Can you tell me when?"

We are rarely trained to give precise answers. I still remember my orientation during the week of April 9, 2018, when Tara Marie, RN, shared these general guidelines:

- If they have moderate to significant declines every 4 to 8 weeks, they have months that can become years.
- If they have moderate to significant declines every 2 to 4 weeks, they have weeks that can become months.
- If they have moderate to significant declines every 7 to 14 days, they have days that can become weeks.
- If they have moderate to significant declines several days per week, they have hours that can become days.
- If they have moderate to significant daily declines, they have minutes, which can become hours.

But what constitutes moderate to significant declines? Are some more significant than others? As a hospice nurse, how can I be more accurate and respond empathetically and compassionately to our patients and their families?

Over the following years, I learned to observe changes and interview caregivers and families. When a patient or family member asks these deeply personal and challenging questions, I can confidently answer them, emphasizing that these are just estimates and only God knows the exact date and time.

This book aims to share the wisdom I've gained over the past several years to help you grow and flourish as a hospice professional.

For caregivers and family members reading this book, I hope you learn what we, as hospice professionals, wish to know to answer your essential questions as accurately as possible. Perhaps you can use the information in this book to answer the question yourself.

To prepare you, the reader, please note that the initial chapters and writings will answer the question of "Are we in the two weeks or less range?" as the book continues, going over the gambit of less than six months, less than three months, etc. The reason for this is that if we are alike, we are hardest hit by missing that our patient is about to die even when a single person did not ask that question.

Chapter 1

The Art of Observing and Interviewing

A New Perspective

I understand that most hospice nurses began their careers in other areas of nursing before entering the beautiful and compassionate field of hospice. Some of you worked in the emergency room, others in intensive care, etc. In those areas, our observational skills were honed to recognize when someone was about to crash (or witnessing it as they arrived), prompting us to respond with a code blue or a request for the rapid response team or by reading lab values and vital signs to recommend specific actions to the provider.

We monitored vital signs and lab values closely; for example, if a patient's oxygen saturation dropped below 91%, we would administer oxygen 2 liters per minute via nasal cannula unless instructed otherwise. If their blood pressure exceeded a certain threshold, there were often standing orders to give 10 mg of hydralazine IV push, and so on.

The focus was on rescuing or saving the patient. Our interviewing skills were tightly focused on PQRST (Provocation, Quality, Region or Radiation, Severity or Scale, and Timing), whether the patient preferred their pills whole or crushed, or background questions like "Do you have any drug allergies?" or "Have you had any previous surgeries?"

In the emergency room, we might have delved into what brought the patient there, while on other hospital floors, we might have asked get-to-know-you questions. However, only some of these questions were geared toward determining specific declines. We all operated within the framework of saving and rescuing; even our skills at noticing subtle declines were essential to keeping the patient alive.

When we enter hospice, we must intentionally rewire our thinking about what matters to those who are terminally ill. Our focus shifts to comfort and encouragement, and we no longer have immediate access to a stock room, utility room, or nearby hospital-based pharmacy. We learn to be resourceful, using our car stock, bag, and individual ingenuity to provide care.

Not only do we have to relearn which vital signs matter under different circumstances, but we also must learn to observe with all our senses and interview the patient, caregivers, and family members.

This book focuses on using these new and constantly refined skills to answer the patient's question, "When will I die?" The skills you are developing will have far-reaching effects, helping you become the best hospice nurse you can be.

Observing with all Our Senses

Did you know death has a smell, and those who are in their last 30 to 45 days of life smell differently than when they were several months away from death? Did you know that frequent changes in one's breathing pattern, going from labored to unlabored or faster to slower, are clues to monitor?

If you've not already been doing this as part of your hospice nursing practice, I want to encourage you to take your time to let everything sink in when you walk into the area where you will meet with and assess your patient. Imagine walking through the forest, trying to see both the forest and the individual trees. Engage all of your senses as they will not only aid you in observing the subtle signs your patient is heading closer to death, but will also help you as you assess for comfort, for medication side effects, and answer other important questions such as "is it the disease process or the medications?"

The interviewing part should include standard questions such as determining the discomfort level vs. comfort, but our senses and critical thinking of what we are smelling, hearing, and seeing should also impact what questions we ask of the patient, caregivers, and family members.

Allow me to give you an example of allowing your senses to be broad and narrow. I was doing the tuck-in visit for a patient who had been transferred from a local skilled nursing facility, where another nurse handled the admission and subsequent visits. This was my first time seeing the patient who would become part of my census.

As I entered the small, cozy home, I immediately saw our patient lying on a hospital bed, surrounded by several family members. I could determine she appeared comfortable via the PAINAD scale immediately due to unlabored breathing, a calm facial expression, and a relaxed body. The one son promptly greeted me and quickly pulled me over to the nearby unenclosed kitchen just a few feet away; I could still see the patient by turning to my right and hearing in that area.

Several family members soon joined the son and me in that small space, asking various questions, including having me review all the medications that came home with the patient from the facility. As I listened to them and responded (being among the trees, so to write), I did not isolate my senses to my immediate surroundings. Still, I carefully listened to the patient's initial rhythmic breathing in the room nearby.

I paused the discussion with the family for approximately 15 minutes when the rhythmic breathing became irregular and labored. Then, based on that new assessment, I noted where we were at with the family discussion items and changed it to that of an interviewer asking questions going over the last 72 hours of their visits with their loved one at the facility, including how things went shortly after EMS dropped the patient home.

The result allowed for the conclusion that the patient was transitioning towards actively dying, and the particular agency for whom I was working included that period for daily visits (some agencies hold daily visits until the patient is actively dying).

I don't share this experience to magnify myself as some of you who may be reading this book have decades of experience, and others just as much as I do. These are not superhuman powers or anything unique to me. I share them from the perspective that if I can do it, so can you. If I can develop the ability to see the trees in front of me and the forest they are within, so can you.

Now, let's dig in deeper.

Why Observational and Interviewing Skills Matter

There are observation and interviewing skills you can develop which will help you learn:

- What could cause the current change in condition
- Determining if a patient is having terminal restlessness
- Determining if your patient is within two weeks or less of life to live
- Knowing where your patient is in the dying process

Anyone with patience and love toward the person being observed and interviewed can hone and develop these skills.

Observation Key Areas

Remember that the skin is the largest organ of the body. As such, it is often the first area to change when we are sick.

- **Complexion**—ashen, pale/pallor, waxy/glossy looking—all of these are signs that the patient has a condition change. If your patient's complexion is none of these, do your best to memorize or take note of their baseline because complexion changes fall into the category of moderate (if they are slightly pale, for example) to significant (ashen) change in condition.
- **Eyes**—is the patient looking at you when you address and talk with them or looking through or past you? Are they seeing beings, objects, and people not present in the room? All of these are indications that the patient is changing mental status.

- **Mottling**—red to purple, marbling/splotchy areas often first found on the patient's feet and legs can indicate the person is within days or less of dying.
- **Is the patient lethargic**—tired on steroids where the patient tries to stay awake but can barely keep their eyes open, talk (may or may not have slurred speech), etc.?
- **Is your patient non-responsive?**
- **Breathing:** Labored vs. unlabored? Rhythmic vs. arrhythmic? Hyperventilating vs. hyperventilating?

All the above can indicate the patient is within two weeks or less of life to live.

Interviewing Key Areas

It is helpful to interview the patient, their loved ones, and any staff (if at a facility). Your goal is to flesh out the following areas:

- Has the patient had any restlessness such as fidgeting, frequent position changes, picking at things not present, appearing to play or interact with objects not present, scratching into their skin without realizing it, or other signs of anxiety? This is to flesh out if a patient is having terminal restlessness.
- To what degree do they need help with the current texture of their food and liquids? Here, you are looking for two things: a medium change where maybe their textures (food and liquid) need to be downgraded for protection against aspiration pneumonia and choking or a notable change such as being told food and liquids are just rolling out of their mouth which is a significant indicator for if your patient is within two weeks or less of life to live.
- Is the patient having periods of severe sweating (diaphoresis), acting, or complaining they are too hot or too cold without regard to the actual temperature in the home, especially if everyone else is comfortable?
- What has the flow of urine been like? Steady, slowing, almost non-existent, and then a splurge out of nowhere? The latter is typically a sign that the body is getting ready to give out; in my experience, this is a sign of cleansing.

- Has the patient had increasing periods of intractable nausea with emesis or loose stools? This can create electrolyte balances, pushing the patient faster towards the end of life.
- Has the patient had increased periods of confusion, including hallucinations? Do any of the hallucinations include people the patient knew that have since died? The latter is a spirit-based sign that the patient may be within the last two weeks to one month of life.
- Has the patient had a burst of energy appearing out of nowhere? This can look like getting up earlier to eat, eating beyond 100% more than usual, being awake far more than expected, and other indicators that make people around the patient question whether they are not terminal (i.e., they are having a rally).
- How fast have the downward changes been taking place? I.e., one medium to significant change every four to six weeks? One medium to significant change every two to four weeks? One medium to significant change per week? Multiple changes per day or week? The more frequent the changes, especially in the last two questions, the more your patient is within two weeks or less of life to live.

Trigger Words

Suppose we hear from the patient or caregivers or read certain words or phrases in the caregiver or facility staff notes. In that case, we should be on high alert for the possibility that the patient is either transitioning towards actively dying or is otherwise close to transitioning. Those trigger words and phrases are as follows:

Sleeping all day: Anywhere from 20 hours to a full day is significant.

Significant Decrease in Food and Fluid Intake: This might manifest as only taking sips of liquid, eating small bites, or refusing food and fluids altogether.

Changes in Consciousness: This includes confusion, disorientation, lethargy, or becoming non-responsive.

Changes in Breathing: Irregular, shallow, or labored breathing can indicate the body's decline.

Picking at Things We Cannot See: Often an early sign of terminal restlessness.

Speaking to or About Departed Loved Ones: Sometimes, patients might start talking to deceased relatives or friends.

Expression of Farewells or Closure: Patients might desire to say goodbye or exhibit behaviors that suggest they are preparing to pass.

Changes in Skin Color and Temperature: The skin may become cool to the touch and take on a pale or mottled appearance.

Pain and Discomfort: An increase in discomfort or pain not effectively managed with medication. The phrase "hurts all over" is typically a significant sign.

Sudden Onset Symptoms

Whether this is revealed during the observation and interview or the actual physical assessment, one of the most noticeable signs that a person may have less than two weeks to live is a sudden onset of symptoms within 72 hours.

- **Generalized discomfort:** The patient may feel pain or discomfort all over their body, even when not touched or moved. They may grimace, moan, or cry out in pain. They may need more pain medication or other comfort measures to ease their suffering.
- **Dysphagia:** The patient may have trouble swallowing pills, food, or liquid. They may choke, cough, or gag when they try to eat or drink. They may lose their appetite or refuse to eat or drink anything. As a result, they may become dehydrated or malnourished.
- **Lethargy:** The patient may become very sleepy, drowsy, or unresponsive. They may not open their eyes, speak, or react to stimuli. They may drift in and out of consciousness or slip into

a coma. They may not recognize their loved ones or their surroundings.

- **Spitting out food or having food appear to roll out of their mouth:** The patient may lose their ability to control their mouth muscles. They may be unable to chew, swallow, or spit out food. They may drool or have food come out of their mouth. They may also have difficulty breathing or clearing their airway.

- **Restlessness and agitation:** The patient may become restless, agitated, or confused. They may move around in bed, pull at their clothes or sheets, or try to get out of bed. They may yell "Help me, help me" or other words or phrases. They may have hallucinations, delusions, or paranoia. They may be experiencing anxiety, fear, or unresolved issues.

- **Skin mottling:** The patient may have patches of purple, blue, or red skin on their hands, feet, arms, or legs. This is caused by poor blood circulation and low oxygen levels. The skin may also feel cold, clammy, or sweaty.

- **Dusky/ashen complexion:** The patient may have a pale, gray, or bluish color on their face, lips, or nails. This is also caused by poor blood circulation and low oxygen levels.

- **Hyperventilation:** The patient may breathe extremely fast, shallow, or irregularly, with more than 24 breaths per minute. They may have Cheyne-Stokes breathing, alternating rapidly and with no breathing periods. They may also have Kussmaul breathing, a pattern of deep, labored breathing. These breathing patterns indicate that the patient's body struggles to maintain normal functions.

- **Multiple falls within 72 hours:** The patient may suddenly lose balance, coordination, or strength. They may fall or collapse when they try to stand up, walk, or move. They may injure themselves or become unconscious as a result. They may have a stroke, a seizure, or a brain hemorrhage.

These symptoms are typically tell-tale signs that, outside of an infection, the disease progression has taken a sudden turn, such that the patient may die at any moment and up to two weeks later. They indicate that the patient's vital organs, such as the heart, lungs, kidneys, liver, and brain, are shutting down and failing. They also indicate that the patient is experiencing a lot of physical and emotional distress and needs more care and support.

Chapter 2

The Assessment

Early Signs vs Late Signs

An early sign of end-of-life typically means the loved one may have up to a month to live, but it is often two weeks or less. Late signs usually mean two weeks or less; some very late signs frequently mean the loved one is in their last three days.

Goldfish breathing, fish-out-of-water breathing, and taking guppy breaths are extremely late signs and critical to be taken seriously in preparing everyone for the last breath.

Significant Findings

Breathing — Cheyne Stokes, Kussmaul, Goldfish breathing, fish-out-of-water breathing, taking guppy breaths (very late sign)—typically indicates less than three days.

Cool extremities (early sign) — are the person's hands cold? Their calves, their feet? — Frigid cold (very late sign — typically indicates less than 36 hours).

Comatose state (late sign) — unresponsive, cannot be awakened?

Cyanosis (varies based on the disease process in terms of early, middle, and late) — Assess cheeks, lips, fingernail beds, toenails, and toes.

Death Rattle (very late sign) — gurgling, gargling sound with breathing (can be an early sign for loved ones who have congestive heart failure).

Ears pinning (early sign) — Pinned ears look like the person has their lower earlobe pinned to their neck. This effect occurs in most people in the last two weeks of life due to a non-suffering form of dehydration.

Eyes glassy, tearing, half-open (late sign) — unable to track or focus on those around the person.

Mottling (late sign, but in some disease processes, can be middle) — their skin looks blotchy or has different colors in patches. It happens because their body is not getting enough blood and oxygen as they near the end of their life.

Restlessness (unless habitual, late sign) — unsettled, frequently changing position, high fall risk.

Temperature deregulation (late sign unless brain cancer or brain injury) — too hot even when it's cool or very cold for others, too cold even when everyone is sweating. Often, it involves taking clothes off and putting clothes or blankets on.

Chapter 3

Observable Signs and Symptoms of Decline

The information you gather from observing and interviewing should be tracked in a HIPAA-compliant manner outside the hospice agency EMR documentation system so you can review and follow the changes in condition over time. Using that information, you can picture the patient's journey through the end of life. The following are broadly painted as to what you might see as the patient progresses through this journey.

Six Months or Less to Live

As a terminal illness progresses, specific changes become more common. Around six months before the end of life, you may notice some of the following signs and symptoms:

- **Decreased Appetite**: The patient might show less interest in eating. They may have difficulty swallowing, chewing, or digesting food. They may also experience nausea, vomiting, or constipation.
- **Fatigue**: They may become increasingly tired and need more rest. They may have less energy and motivation to do things. They may also have difficulty breathing, especially when lying down.
- **Weight Loss**: Significant loss of body weight over the past few months. This can be due to decreased appetite, increased metabolism, or muscle wasting. This can make them look thinner, weaker, and frailer. It can also affect their immune system and increase their risk of infections and complications.
- **Physical Decline**: A decline in their overall physical abilities and activities. They may have more pain, discomfort, or symptoms related to their illness. They may also have

difficulty moving, walking, or performing daily tasks. They may need more assistance and care from you or others.

- **Increased Sleep**: Spending more time sleeping or in bed (12 to 16 hours per day is typical). They may also become less alert, responsive, or coherent when awake. They may struggle to recognize you or others, remember things, or make decisions. They may also experience confusion, hallucinations, or delusions. This can be due to changes in their brain function, medication side effects, or lack of oxygen.

Three Months or Less to Live

As the illness advances, these signs and symptoms may become more pronounced:

- **Pain**: Physical discomfort may increase, leading to grimacing, fidgeting, or moaning. This can be due to the progression of the disease, inflammation, infection, or pressure on the nerves or organs. Pain can affect the person's mood, sleep, and quality of life.
- **Emotional Distress**: Feelings of nervousness, anxiety, or confusion might arise. This can be due to the fear of death, the loss of control, the uncertainty of the future, or the changes in brain function. Emotional distress can affect a person's behavior, communication, and relationships.
- **Withdrawal**: People might become less engaged with others and more focused inward. This can be due to loss of interest, lack of energy, or preparation for death. Withdrawal can affect the person's social and spiritual needs.
- **Restlessness**: Agitation and restlessness could become more noticeable. This can be due to discomfort, anxiety, confusion, or unresolved issues. Restlessness can affect the person's safety, comfort, and peace of mind.
- **Sleeping more**: Sleeping and napping are 14 to 18 hours daily. This can be due to fatigue, medication, or the body shutting down. Sleeping more can affect the person's awareness, responsiveness, and communication.

One Month or Less to Live

In the final weeks, you may observe:

- **Cognitive Changes**: A decrease in cognitive ability and concentration. This can be due to the reduced blood flow to the brain, medication effects, or metabolic changes. Cognitive changes can affect a person's memory, judgment, logic, and awareness.
- **Changes in Breathing**: Breathing patterns may become irregular or more labored due to fluid buildup in the lungs, weakness of the respiratory muscles, or pressure on the chest. Breathing changes can affect the person's oxygen level, comfort, and anxiety.
- **Hallucinations**: Visions or hallucinations might occur. This can be due to changes in brain function, medication effects, or spiritual experiences. Hallucinations can affect a person's perception, emotion, and communication.
- **Loss of Appetite**: Appetite further diminishes. This can be due to the reduced need for food and fluids, difficulty swallowing or digesting, or loss of taste or smell. Loss of appetite can affect the person's hydration, nutrition, and comfort
- **Skin Changes**: Skin temperature and color may fluctuate. This can be due to poor circulation, reduced blood pressure, or organ failure. Skin changes can affect the person's warmth, sensation, and appearance.
- **Sleeping more**: Sleeping and napping are around 20+ hours daily. This can be due to exhaustion, medication effects, or the body shutting down. Sleeping more can affect the person's awareness, responsiveness, and communication

Two Weeks or Less to Live

In the last two weeks, the following changes might occur:

- **Inactivity**: Decreased activity and loss of function. This can be due to weakness, fatigue, or paralysis of the muscles and

nerves. Inactivity can affect a person's mobility, posture, and comfort.
- **Communication**: Difficulty talking and expressing thoughts. This can be due to reduced blood flow to the brain, dryness in the mouth, or weakness in the vocal cords. Communication can affect a person's cognition, emotion, and interaction.
- **Congestion**: Congestion in the lungs or throat could lead to changes in breathing. This can be due to the accumulation of mucus, saliva, or blood in the airways, the infection or inflammation of the lungs, or the relaxation of the throat muscles. Congestion can affect the person's oxygen level, comfort, and sound.
- **Sleeping more**: Sleeping and napping occur for 22+ hours daily. This can be due to exhaustion, medication effects, or the body shutting down. Sleeping more can affect a person's awareness, responsiveness, and communication.

Last Days of Life

In the final days, expect:

- **Withdrawal from the External World**: Increased isolation and disengagement. This can be due to loss of interest, lack of energy, or preparation for death. Withdrawal from the external world can affect the person's social and spiritual needs.
- **Loss of Appetite**: Appetite may cease entirely. This can be due to the reduced need for food and fluids, difficulty swallowing or digesting, or loss of taste or smell. Loss of appetite can affect the person's hydration, nutrition, and comfort.
- **Change in Bowel and Bladder Functions**: Bowel and bladder functions may change. This can be due to the decreased intake of food and fluids, the reduced activity of the digestive system, or the loss of muscle control. Changes in bowel and bladder functions can affect the person's hygiene, comfort, and dignity
- **Confusion**: Confusion and disorientation could become more prominent. This can be due to the reduced blood flow to the

brain, medication effects, or metabolic changes. Confusion can affect the person's memory, judgment, logic, and awareness

- **Visions**: Visions and hallucinations might occur. This can be due to changes in brain function, medication effects, or spiritual experiences. Visions can affect a person's perception, emotion, and communication.
- **Sleeping more**: Sleeping and napping are around 23+ hours daily without waking up. This can be due to exhaustion, medication effects, or the body shutting down. Sleeping more can affect a person's awareness, responsiveness, and communication. You can help them by making them comfortable, adjusting their position, and keeping them clean and dry.

Chapter 4

Using the Palliative Performance Scale

Palliative Performance Scale (PPSv2) version 2[2]					
PPS Level	Ambulation	Activity & Evidence of Disease	Self-Care	Intake	Conscious Level
100%	Full	Normal activity & work No evidence of disease	Full	Normal	Full
90%	Full	Normal activity & work Some evidence of disease	Full	Normal	Full
80%	Full	Normal activity with effort Some evidence of disease	Full	Normal or reduced	Full
70%	Reduced	Unable to do normal job/work Significant disease	Full	Normal or reduced	Full
60%	Reduced	Unable to do hobby/housework Significant disease	Occasional assistance necessary	Normal or reduced	Full or confusion
50%	Mainly sit/lie	Unable to do any work Extensive disease	Considerable assistance required	Normal or reduced	Full or confusion
40%	Mainly in bed	Unable to do most activity Extensive disease	Mainly assistance	Normal or reduced	Full or drowsy +/- confusion
30%	Totally bed bound	Unable to do any activity Extensive disease	Total care	Normal or reduced	Full or drowsy +/- confusion
20%	Totally bed bound	Unable to do any activity Extensive disease	Total care	Minimal to sips	Full or drowsy +/- confusion
10%	Totally bed bound	Unable to do any activity Extensive disease	Total care	Mouth care only	Drowsy or coma +/- confusion
0%	Death	-	-	-	-

Stable: 100%–80% | Transitional: 70%–40% | End-of-Life: 30%–0%

The Palliative Performance Scale (PPS) can estimate a patient's life expectancy. This functional assessment tool should be coupled with your observations, interviews, and notes of the moderate to significant declines you have documented.

Let's examine what we will see as the PPS changes throughout our patient's end-of-life journey. We can estimate the time left based on the following landmarks and progressions discussed below:

Approximately six months from death

- **High Functioning:** At the start of month six, patients often have higher PPS scores, indicating relatively better functional abilities. This means they can still do many things alone, such as walking, eating, dressing, and bathing. They may also be able to participate in activities they enjoy, such as reading, watching TV, or spending time with family and friends.

Approximately five months from death

- **Gradual Decline:** PPS scores might gradually decline by this point, indicating decreased functional abilities. This means they may need more help with tasks like getting in and out of bed, using the bathroom, or taking medications. They may also have more symptoms, such as pain, fatigue, nausea, or shortness of breath. They may also lose interest in some activities or have trouble concentrating or remembering things.
- **Symptom Management:** Focus on symptom management and addressing discomfort to ensure patients' comfort and well-being. Assess their symptoms regularly and use medications, therapies, or other interventions to relieve them. Monitor their vital signs, such as blood pressure, pulse, temperature, and oxygen level. Check for signs of infection, bleeding, or other complications and report them to the hospice team.
- **Support:** Provide emotional support to patients and families as they navigate these changes. Acknowledge their feelings and validate them. Reassure them that they are not alone and that you are there to help them. Use relaxation techniques, counseling, or spiritual care to help them cope with stress, anxiety, or depression. Respect their values, beliefs, and wishes to help them maintain their sense of dignity, identity, and purpose.

Approximately four months from death

- **Further Decline:** PPS scores may continue to decrease, reflecting a more significant decline in functional status. This means they may become more dependent on caregivers for most tasks, such as eating, drinking, or personal hygiene. They may also have more severe symptoms, such as pain, confusion, agitation, or hallucinations. They may also have changes in their appearance, such as weight loss, skin breakdown, or swelling.

- **Comfort Care:** Prioritize comfort care measures, such as pain management and psychosocial support, to enhance the quality of life. You should use medications, therapies, or other interventions to control pain and other symptoms. It would be best to use comfort measures, such as massage, music, aromatherapy, or touch, to soothe and calm them. To promote relaxation, you should also provide a comfortable and peaceful environment, such as adjusting the lighting, temperature, or noise level.
- **Education:** Educate families about the progressive nature of the disease and the importance of holistic care. You should explain what to expect in the coming weeks and months and how to prepare for them. It would be best if you also taught them how to provide care to the patient, such as how to turn, position, or lift them, prevent bedsores or infections, or administer medications or treatments. It would be best to inform them about the available resources and services they can access, such as respite care, bereavement support, or financial assistance.

Approximately three months from death

- **Greater Dependence:** Due to declining functional abilities, patients might become more dependent on caregivers. This means they may need constant care and supervision, such as feeding, changing, or bathing. They may also have difficulty communicating, such as speaking, hearing, or understanding. They may also have limited awareness, such as recognizing people, places, or time.
- **Holistic Approach:** Adopt a holistic approach to care, addressing physical, emotional, and spiritual needs. Treat the patient as a whole person, not just a disease. Respect their individuality, personality, and history. Honor their culture, religion, and traditions. Help them find meaning, hope, and peace.

- **Caregiver Support:** Offer support and resources to caregivers, recognizing their vital role in the patient's journey. Acknowledging their efforts, challenges, and sacrifices would be best. You should also appreciate their strengths, skills, and knowledge. You should also help them balance their and the patient's needs, such as taking breaks, getting enough sleep, eating well, or exercising. You should also help them cope with their emotions, such as guilt, anger, or grief, by providing counseling, support groups, or spiritual care.

Approximately two months from death

- **Limited Mobility:** PPS scores may indicate limited mobility and self-care abilities. This means they may be bedridden or chair-bound, requiring assistance for all movements. They may also have impaired vision, hearing, or taste. They may also have reduced appetite, thirst, or bowel and bladder function.
- **Personalized Care:** This is the cornerstone of end-of-life care. Tailoring care plans to each patient's unique needs and preferences is crucial in promoting dignity and comfort. It's essential to ask them what they want and don't want, such as medications, treatments, or interventions. Respecting their choices and decisions is paramount, even if they differ from yours or the medical teams. Involving them in their care as much as possible, such as asking for their consent, feedback, or suggestions, is vital to this process.
- **Advance Care Planning:** As a healthcare provider, you are crucial in advance care planning. Engage in discussions to ensure patient wishes are respected. You are responsible for discussing patients' goals, values, and beliefs regarding end-of-life care and helping them complete advance directives. You can communicate patients' wishes to the hospice team and other healthcare providers.

Approximately one month from death

- **Critical Stage:** Patients with significantly reduced functional abilities may reach a critical stage. This means they may have minimal or no response to stimuli, such as sound, touch, or pain. They may also have irregular breathing, pulse, or blood pressure. Recognizing signs of impending death, such as mottled skin, cold extremities, or Cheyne-Stokes respiration, is crucial at this stage.
- **Focus on Comfort:** Shifting the focus entirely to comfort and quality of life in the final stages is a compassionate approach to end-of-life care. Minimizing interventions with limited benefits and discontinuing any medications, treatments, or procedures that are not essential or effective can help ensure the patient's comfort. Avoiding any actions that may cause discomfort or distress, such as moving, suctioning, or testing, and providing comfort measures, such as moistening the mouth, applying lip balm, or elevating the head to ease discomfort, demonstrates a deep sense of empathy and care for the patient.
- **Family Engagement:** Your role in involving families in decision-making and providing emotional support is significant. Informing them of the patient's condition, prognosis, and what to expect in the final days and hours is crucial to your role. Respecting their wishes and preferences regarding the place and manner of death is another aspect of your support. Helping them say goodbye and express their love and gratitude to the patient and preparing them for the death and the aftermath is a crucial part of your support.

Any acute changes to PPS, especially when the change is significant, should involve the critical question: Is this person in the last two weeks, or is there a reversible event that we need to investigate promptly?

Chapter 5

Eating and Sleeping

Eating

When someone is close to dying, they may sleep increasingly more. This is because their body is resting and preparing for the final transition. This is normal and not something to worry about. They may not want to eat or drink much when they are awake. This is also normal and part of the dying process. They may only need a few bites or sips to keep them comfortable. Here is how much food they may need based on how long they are awake:

- If awake for 8 to 12 hours a day, they may need about half or a little more of the food they usually ate when they were healthy.
- If awake 6 to 10 hours a day, they may need about 40-50% of the food they usually eat.
- If awake for 4 to 6 hours a day, they may need about 30-40% of the food they usually eat.
- If awake for 1 to 2 hours a day, they may need about 20-30% of the food they usually eat.

Estimated Time Left	Estimated Calories Needed per Day
Less than six months	1,200 to 1,500 per day
Less than three months	1,000 to 1,200 per day
Less than one month	800 to 1,000 per day
Less than two weeks	600 to 800 per day
The last week of life	Energy needs are minimal.

Another factor that affects how much food the terminally ill patient needs is how long they are awake during the day. Here is how much food they may need based on how long they are awake:

- If awake for 8 to 12 hours a day, they may need about half or a little more of the food they usually ate when they were healthy.
- If awake 6 to 10 hours a day, they may need about 40-50% of the food they usually eat.
- If awake for 4 to 6 hours a day, they may need about 30-40% of the food they usually eat.
- If awake for 1 to 2 hours a day, they may need about 20-30% of the food they usually eat.

Hours Awake	Estimated Calories Needed per Day
8 to 12 hours daily	1,000 to 1,200 per day
6 to 8 hours daily	800 to 1,000 per day
4 to 6 hours daily	600 to 800 per day
1 to 2 hours daily	Energy needs are minimal.

The patient's activity level also determines caloric needs.

- If they can walk around the house a little bit, they may need about 10-15% of the food they usually ate when they were healthy.
- If they can only move from the bed to the chair and back, they may need about 5-10% of the food they usually eat.
- If they cannot get out of bed, they may need only 1-5% of the food they usually eat.

Activity Level	Estimated Calories Needed per Day
Walking around the house	600 to 800 per day
Living a bed-to-chair existence	400 to 600 per day
Bedbound	200 to 400 per day

By tracking your patient's intake, you can better gauge moderate to significant decline, which will be discussed in the next chapter.

Sleeping

Chapter 3 mentions different ranges of sleeping time based on decline. Let us now look at a summary:

Hours Sleeping	Estimated Time Left
12 to 16	Less than six months
14 to 18	Less than three months
20 to 21	Less than one month
22+	Two weeks or less

Everyone is different, and the author points out that sleep time should be combined with other indicators for a more complete picture.

Chapter 6

Understanding Functional Decline

In the introduction of this book, I provided the general guidelines I was given to gauge when a terminally ill person may die.

- If they have moderate to significant declines every 4 to 8 weeks, they have months that can become years.
- If they have moderate to significant declines every 2 to 4 weeks, they have weeks that can become months.
- If they have moderate to significant declines every 7 to 14 days, they have days that can become weeks.
- If they have moderate to significant declines several days per week, they have hours that can become days.
- If they have moderate to significant daily declines, they have minutes, which can become hours.

But what is a moderate decline compared to a significant decline?

Examples of Moderate to Significant Decline

As a person approaches the end of life, their body and mind may undergo various changes affecting their functioning and well-being. These changes can be moderate or significant, depending on how much they interfere with the person's normal activities and comfort. Some examples of moderate and significant declines are:

Moderate Declines

- **Alzheimer's Progression:** Alzheimer's disease is a type of dementia that causes memory loss and cognitive impairment. It has seven stages, from mild to severe. A moderate decline in Alzheimer's is when a person moves from stage 7A to stage 7B, which means they lose the ability to speak or smile and need assistance with all essential tasks.

- **Eating Habits:** Eating is essential for maintaining health and energy. A moderate decline in eating habits is when a person who used to eat full meals now eats less than half of what they used to. This can be due to loss of appetite, difficulty swallowing, nausea, pain, or depression.
- **Oxygen Requirements:** Oxygen is vital for the functioning of the organs and tissues. A moderate decline in oxygen requirements is when a person who could breathe normally now needs supplemental oxygen at night or during the day. This can be due to lung disease, heart failure, or low blood pressure.
- **Mobility:** Mobility is the ability to move around and perform physical activities. A moderate decline in mobility is when a person who could walk without help now needs a cane or a walker. This can be due to muscle weakness, joint pain, balance problems, or fatigue.
- **Frequent Falls:** Falls are a common cause of injury and disability among older adults. A moderate decline in fall frequency is when a person who rarely falls now falls every one or two weeks. This can be due to vision problems, medication side effects, dizziness, or confusion.
- **Dietary Changes:** Diet is the type and amount of food a person eats. A moderate diet decline occurs when a person who could eat regular food now needs softer food that is easier to chew and swallow. This can be due to dental problems, dry mouth, or swallowing difficulties.
- **Orientation Shift:** Orientation is the awareness of oneself and one's surroundings. A moderate decline in orientation is when a person who was fully oriented to person, place, time, and situation now becomes confused about one of these aspects, usually time. This can be due to dementia, delirium, or medication effects.
- **Complexion Alteration:** Complexion is the color and texture of the skin. A moderate decline in complexion is when a person with a healthy skin tone becomes pale yellow or shows subtle changes. This can be due to liver problems, anemia, or dehydration.

- **Sleep Patterns:** Sleep is the state of rest and recovery for the body and mind. A moderate decline in sleep patterns is when a person who used to sleep eight to twelve hours a day, including naps, now sleeps twelve to sixteen hours a day. This can be due to depression, pain, or reduced activity.

Significant Declines

- **Advanced Alzheimer's:** A significant decline in Alzheimer's is when a person jumps from stage 7A to stage 7C or later, which means they lose the ability to respond to their environment, control their movements, or recognize their loved ones.
- **Severe Eating Decline:** A significant decline in eating habits is when a person who used to eat full meals stops eating. This can be due to severe nausea, pain, or loss of consciousness.
- **Continuous Oxygen:** A significant decline in oxygen requirements occurs when a person who needs supplemental oxygen occasionally needs it continuously. This can be due to respiratory failure, cardiac arrest, or shock.
- **Complete Immobility:** A significant decline in mobility is when a person who can walk with assistance becomes completely bedridden. This can be due to paralysis, coma, or severe weakness.
- **Frequent Falls:** A significant decline in fall frequency is when a person who fell every one or two weeks now falls one or more times a day. This can be due to severe vision problems, medication overdose, seizures, or strokes.
- **Dietary Shift:** A significant diet decline occurs when a person who could eat softer food now needs pureed food that is easier to swallow. This can be due to severe dental problems, mouth sores, or choking risks.
- **Disorientation:** A significant decline in orientation is when a person is confused about one aspect of their situation and becomes entirely disoriented about the person, place, time, and situation. This can be due to advanced dementia, severe delirium, or brain damage.
- **Complexion Changes:** A significant decline in complexion is when a person who has a pale yellow or subtle skin tone

now becomes dusky, gray, yellow, pale, or waxy. This can be due to organ failure, infection, bleeding, or death.

- **Excessive Sleep:** A significant decline in sleep patterns is when a person who used to sleep twelve to sixteen hours a day now sleeps more than twenty hours a day. This can be due to coma, sedation, or imminent death.

The speed and extent of these declines can vary from person to person, depending on their illness, age, and other factors. However, they can help clinicians estimate how much time is left for the person before they die. They can also help caregivers prepare for the end of life and provide their loved ones with the best possible care and comfort.

Chapter 7

When Might They Die?

Creating a Rough Estimate

Assessing the patient's journey toward the end involves considering the pace of condition changes. When someone is extremely sick and cannot get better, they may start to show some signs that they are getting closer to death. These signs can help us estimate how much time they have left to live. Different people may have other signs, but there are some common ones that we can look for.

One of the signs is how fast their condition changes. This means how often they have new or old problems get worse. For example, they may have more pain, lose more weight, sleep more, or eat less. These changes can tell us which stage of their dying process. Here's a simplified breakdown:

1. **Early Stages (Approximately 6 Months or More Away):** This is when the changes are slow and not very noticeable. They may happen every month or two. The person may still do things they used to do, like talking, walking, or reading. They may have some good and bad days, but they are not getting much worse.
2. **Approaching the End (Around 3 to 6 Months):** This is when the changes are more noticeable and happen more often. They may happen every few weeks. The person may start to have more problems with their body, like breathing, swallowing, or going to the bathroom. They may need more help from others to do things. They may also have more changes in their mood, like feeling sad, angry, or scared.
3. **Nearing the End (About 1 to 3 Months):** This is when the changes are fast and happen frequently. They may happen every week or even every day. The person may have more

severe problems with their body, like infections, bleeding, or organ failure. They may not be able to do anything by themselves. They may also have more changes in their mind, like seeing or hearing things that are not there, forgetting things, or not knowing where they are.

4. **Imminent Death (Less Than 2 Weeks):** This is when the changes are swift and very big. They may happen several times a week or even several times a day. The person's body is getting ready to stop working. They may have low blood pressure, slow heartbeat, shallow breathing, or cold skin. They may be unable to talk, open their eyes, or respond to anything.

What I'm typically assessing on a hospice admission with discussion among the patient and loved ones is as follows:

In the last 30 days

- Increased episodes of generalized pain (hurts all over even to gentle touch) or shortness of breath as evidenced by fast, shallow breathing along with the dates of those events.
- How many falls, and what are the dates of each fall?
- How many infections took place, and what were the dates of those infections?
- How often was the patient lethargic, and what were the dates?
- Has the patient had a new onset of restlessness, agitation, or behavior changes unrelated to an infection? If yes, the dates.
- Did the patient experience any changes to mental status outside of lethargy? If yes, please provide the dates of those changes.
- How many downward changes to functionality, including activities of daily living (ambulating, feeding themselves, dressing, personal hygiene, continence, toileting)? How close are these changes to one another?
- How often did the patient experience dysphagia by date and dietary changes by date?
- How much weight loss?

- Are there any other changes, including treatments that stopped working, worsening vital signs, etc.? Please provide dates for each.

In the last two weeks

- Do you believe there was a whirlwind of downward changes? If so, tell me more.

Assessment Thoughts and Actions Based on a 30-day Review

- If there are daily changes (including several times per day) or several changes per week, the patient is EOL-appropriate, as death may be imminent.
- If the patient has only one change every seven to ten days, the patient should be reassessed for EOL status every visit.
- If the patient has one change every other week, the patient should be assessed for EOL status weekly.

And if they are not that close, then how close?

This involves tracking the downward changes and referring to the table below for a general idea of when.

Frequency of Change	Typically Means Death Within
Once every 4 to 8 weeks	Less than six months
Every 3 to 4 weeks	Less than three months
Every 1 to 2 weeks	Less than two months
Once every week	Less than one month
Several times per week	Less than two weeks
Several times per day	Less than 72 hours
Every minute to every hour	Less than 24 hours

Chapter 8

The Dying Process at the End of Life

While the preceding chapters have focused on estimating when someone might pass away, it's essential to recognize that newer hospice nurses, caregivers, and family members may not fully understand the entire death and dying process. This chapter aims to bridge that gap by providing a compassionate and comprehensive overview.

Living is a continuum. Scientifically, life begins at conception and progresses through various stages—from birth to childhood, adolescence, and adulthood. Throughout these stages, we live actively, often without considering the quality of life. As we approach the end of life, we enter a transitioning phase before actively dying.

This chapter will explore the dying process at the end of life, addressing common questions such as, "What is transitioning?" "How do I know if my loved one is actively dying?" and "What are the phases of dying?" The dying process can be divided into two main phases: transitioning and actively dying.

The Transitioning Phase

This phase marks the beginning of the dying process and can be confusing for loved ones. During this time, the person may still be eating, talking, or even somewhat mobile. This phase can last from a few seconds in sudden events like a heart attack to several weeks.

Signs that your loved one is transitioning include:

- Increased restlessness, which may indicate terminal restlessness.

- Subtle changes in complexion, becoming more pronounced as they near active dying. This may appear as pallor, greyness, or flushing.
- Reports of seeing and speaking to deceased loved ones.
- Spending more time alone, napping, or sleeping.
- Significant reduction in food intake over days or weeks.
- Noticeable changes in breathing patterns—faster, slower, or irregular.
- Periods of fixed staring, where they seem to look through you rather than at you.
- Loss of mobility and difficulty repositioning themselves.
- Trouble eating due to a weakening gag reflex.

As your loved one spends more time sleeping and showing these changes, they are likely nearing the end of the transitioning phase and moving into the actively dying stage.

The Actively Dying Phase

The active dying phase begins when your loved one becomes unconscious. Even experienced healthcare professionals may find it challenging to pinpoint the exact transition from the transitioning phase to active dying. Some professionals simplify this by informing families that their loved one is dying, thus combining the two phases.

Key characteristics of the actively dying phase include:

- They may be in a comatose-like state, often passing away in their sleep.
- The gag reflex is absent, so avoid giving food or drink to prevent choking.
- More noticeable changes in complexion.
- Respirations become a critical indicator, with patterns that may be extremely fast, slow, or fluctuating.
- Heart rate may become very fast or irregular.
- Ears may pin back, and earlobes may appear close to the neck.
- Development of a terminal fever that is resistant to medication.
- The presence of death gurgles due to accumulated secretions in the airway. This is not painful for them and can be managed

by elevating the head of the bed and using prescribed medications.
- Possible mottling of the extremities due to circulatory changes.
- Unpreventable pressure injuries on bony areas like elbows, hips, knees, and tailbone.
- A significant amount of urine or a bowel movement may occur as the body prepares for the end.

In the final moments, their breathing will become more erratic. Secretions may emerge from their mouth, and they will take their last breath, which may sound like a gasp. This marks the end of their journey.

The Last Hours

Losing a loved one is profoundly difficult and sorrowful. You may wonder how much time they have left and how you can help them. You might also want to say goodbye and express your love. Some signs indicate your loved one is in their final hours, which can help you prepare.

Breathing Changes

In the last 24 to 36 hours, breathing patterns may change. They may breathe faster or slower, deeper or shallower, or stop and start. This is due to the weakening of their body and lungs. Gurgling or rattling sounds may occur because of excess saliva or mucus. You can help by raising your head, wiping your mouth, or offering ice chips.

Rapid Breathing

If breathing becomes very fast, with less than three minutes between breaths, the patient may have less than 12 hours left. Their heart may be beating fast, and their blood pressure may drop. Cold or blue hands and feet indicate poor blood circulation. They may be unable to talk or move due to a lack of oxygen to the brain. Comfort them by holding their hand, speaking softly, or playing soothing music.

Last Breath

When they take their last breath, they may cough or expel saliva or mucus. This is normal and not painful. Reflex breaths may occur after the heart stops as the body shuts down. Check their pulse or listen to their chest to confirm they have passed. Then, say your goodbyes and thank them for being part of your life.

Understanding these phases and signs can help you navigate this challenging time with compassion and preparedness.

Concluding Remarks

Thank you for buying this book, for which I hope you and those for whom you care benefited from the wisdom and experience within it.

I aim to help my fellow nurses, caregivers, and family members grow and learn even in their darkest hours.

Resources

Gone from My Sight: The Dying Experience by Barbara Karnes RN –
A pamphlet that every hospice worker and family member of a
terminally ill loved one should read, available at
https://www.amazon.com/gp/product/B00072HSCY

The Eleventh Hour: A Caring Guideline for the Hours to Minutes
Before Death at https://www.amazon.com/Eleventh-Hour-Caring-
Guideline-Minutes/dp/B002MYGYUW

By Your Side, A Guide for Caring for the Dying at Home at
https://www.amazon.com/Your-Side-Guide-Caring-
Dying/dp/173705681X

PAINAD Assessment Resources at
https://compassioncrossing.info/tag/painad/

The D.O.G.I. At The Window Case Study at
https://compassioncrossing.info/the-d-o-g-i-at-the-window-case-
study/

Delirium vs. terminal Restlessness at
https://compassioncrossing.info/delirium-vs-terminal-restlessness/

Understanding Terminal Restlessness at
https://compassioncrossing.info/understanding-terminal-restlessness/

Clues For Terminal Restlessness Often Missed For Facility Patients at
https://compassioncrossing.info/clues-for-terminal-restlessness-often-
missed-for-facility-patients/

Terminal Restlessness In The Completely Nonverbal Patient at
https://compassioncrossing.info/terminal-restlessness-in-the-
completely-nonverbal-patient/

Author Bio

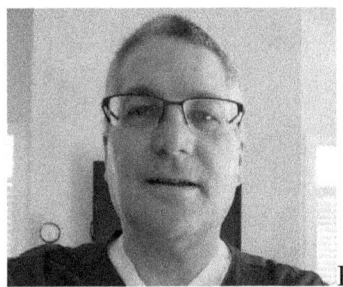

Peter Abraham, BSN, RN is an experienced nurse dedicated to supporting nurses, caregivers, families, and patients in their learning, growth, and well-being journey. Peter's nursing path encompasses practical experience as a cardiac telemetry nurse in a bustling cardiology unit at a Magnet-awarded teaching hospital. Additionally, Peter has fulfilled the role of a second-shift RN supervisor, overseeing an entire building in an SNF/LTC (Skilled Nursing Facility/Long-Term Care) setting with 151 residents. Remarkably, during the initial wave of COVID-19, the facility achieved an impressive close-to-100% recovery rate before operation warp speed was complete.

Furthermore, Peter's nursing career extends to rural home hospice care. As a visiting hospice registered nurse case manager, he offers compassionate care to patients in various settings, including private homes, personal care homes, assisted living facilities, skilled nursing facilities, and hospitals.

Moreover, Peter's desire to help others extends beyond his physical presence. At CompassionCrossing.Info, he writes articles to empower caregivers, family members, and fellow nurses in end-of-life care. Peter's drive to help others, which flows from his love of Christ Jesus, is a source of support and encouragement for all he reaches.

Other books by Peter Abraham include the following:

Empowering Excellence in Hospice: A Nurse's Toolkit for Best Practices series:

Compliance-based, Eligibility Driven Hospice
Documentation: Tips for Hospice Nurses
Whispers of Time: Understanding the End-of-Life Timeline
Terminal Clarity: Hospice Eligibility Guide for Nurses
Mastering Recertifications: A Comprehensive Guide for
Nurses

Compassionate Caregiving series:

Daily Hospice Care Planner: Organize, Communicate, and
Provide Consistent Care
Dignity in Dying: A Thoughtful Approach to Voluntary
Stopping Eating and Drinking
Palliative Sedation: A Compassionate Approach
Hospice Medication Handbook: A Caregiver's Guide to
Comfort Medications
Nourishing Hope: A Caregiver's Guide to End-of-Life
Nutrition
Validation and Compassion: A Guide to Connecting with
Terminally Ill Loved Ones

Dementia Caregivers Essentials series:

Dementia Caregiver Essentials (all ten books below in one)

Anger Management in Dementia
CPAP and Oxygen for Dementia
Diabetes Care for Dementia
Hallucination Management for Dementia
Infection Awareness in Dementia
Medication Compliance for Dementia
Music Therapy for Dementia
Nutrition for Dementia
Placement for Dementia
Sundowning Management for Dementia

Holistic Nurse: Skills for Excellence series

Dementia Staging Mastery: A Nurse's Guide to Dementia Assessment

The above books can be found on Amazon at
https://amzn.to/3YFBYQ0

Connect with Peter On:

Website: https://compassioncrossing.info/